ANCIENT EGYPT OPHTHALMOLOGY

THE EYE

Dr.Alaaeldin Hamada

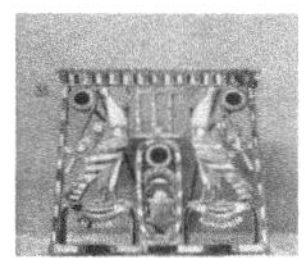

ISBN: 9798577935337

Cover design by: Art Painter
Library of Congress Control Number: 2018675309
Printed in the United States of America

*I dedicate this book to Imhotep "the great master " ,and also my
master who i never met but in his books ; Dr.Paul Ghalioungui .
dedication to future minds which recognise the ultimate
importance of ancient egyptian practice in all fields .
special dedication to my love ; zainab ,who believed in
me and pushed me to continue this project.*

CONTENTS

INTRODUCTION

The medicine of the ancient Egyptians is some of the oldest documented. From the beginnings of the civilization in the late fourth millennium BC until the Persian invasion of 525 BC, Egyptian medical practice went largely unchanged but was highly advanced for its time, including simple non-invasive surgery, setting of bones, dentistry, and an extensive set of pharmacopoeia. Egyptian medical thought influenced later traditions, including the Greeks.

Until the 19th century, the main sources of information about ancient Egyptian medicine were writings from later in antiquity. In 1822, the translation of the Rosetta stone finally allowed the translation of ancient Egyptian hieroglyphic inscriptions and papyri, including many related to medical matters (Egyptian medical papyri). The resultant interest in Egyptology in the 19th century led to the discovery of several sets of extensive ancient medical documents, including the Ebers papyrus, the Edwin Smith Papyrus, the Hearst Papyrus, the London Medical Papyrus and others dating back as far as 2900 BC.

The Edwin Smith Papyrus is a textbook on surgery and details anatomical observations and the "examination, diagnosis, treatment, and prognosis" of numerous ailments. It was probably written around 1600 BC, but is regarded as a copy of several earlier texts. Medical information in it dates from as early as 3000 BC. It is thus viewed as a learning manual. Treatments consisted of ointments made from animal, vegetable or fruit substances or minerals. There is evidence of oral surgery being performed as early as the 4th Dynasty (2900–2750 BC).

The Ebers papyrus (c. 1550 BC) includes 877 prescriptions – as categorized by a modern editor – for a variety of ailments and illnesses, some of them involving magical remedies, for Egyptian beliefs regarding magic and medicine were often intertwined. It also contains documentation revealing awareness of tumors, along with instructions on tumor removal.

The Kahun Gynaecological Papyrus treats women's complaints, including problems with conception. Thirty four cases detailing diagnosis and treatment survive, some of them fragmentarily. [Dating to 1800 BC, it is the oldest surviving medical text of any kind.

Other documents such as the Hearst papyrus (1450 BC), and Berlin Papyrus (1200 BC) also provide valuable insight into ancient Egyptian medicine.

Other information comes from the images that often adorn the walls of Egyptian tombs and the translation of the accompanying inscriptions. Advances in modern medical technology also contributed to the understanding of ancient Egyptian medicine. Paleopathologists were able to use X-Rays and later CAT Scans to view the bones and organs of mummies. Electron microscopes, mass spectrometry and various forensic techniques allowed scientists unique glimpses of the state of health in Egypt 4000 years ago.

The ancient Egyptians were at least partially aware of the importance of diet, both in balance and moderation. Owing to Egypt's great endowment of fertile land, food production was never a major issue, although, no matter how bountiful the land, paupers and starvation still exist. The main crops for most of ancient Egyptian history were emmer wheat and barley. Consumed in the form of loaves which were produced in a variety of types through baking and fermentation, with yeast greatly enriching the nutritional value of the product, one farmer's crop could support an estimated twenty adults. Barley was also used in beer. Vegetables and fruits of many types were widely grown. Oil was produced from the linseed plant and there was a limited selection of spices and herbs. Meat (sheep, goats, pigs) was regularly available to at least the upper classes and fish were widely consumed, although there is evidence of prohibitions during certain periods against certain types of animal products; Herodotus wrote of the pig as being 'unclean'. Offerings to King Unas (c. 2494–2345 BC) were recorded as "...milk, three kinds of beer, five kinds of wine, ten loaves, four of bread, ten of cakes four meats, different cuts, joints, roast, spleen, limb, breast, quail, goose, pigeon, figs, ten other fruits, three kinds of corn, barley, spelt, five kinds of oil, and fresh plants..."

It is clear that the Egyptian diet was not lacking for the upper classes and that even the lower classes may have had some selection (Nunn, 2002).

Like many civilizations in the past, the ancient Egyptians amply discovered the medicinal properties of plant life around them. In the Edwin Smith Papyrus there are many recipes to help heal different ailments. In a small section of this papyrus, there are five recipes one dealing with problems women may have had, three on techniques for refining the complexion, and the fifth recipe for ailments that deal with the colon. The ancient Egyptians were known to use honey as medicine, and the juices of pomegranates served as both an astringent and a delicacy. In the Ebers Papyrus, there are over 800 remedies; some were topical like ointments, and wrappings, others were oral medication such as pills and mouth rinses;still others were taken through inhalation.: The recipes to cure constipation consisted of berries from the castor oil tree, Male Palm, and Gengent beans, just to name a few. One recipe that was to help headaches called for "inner-of-onion, fruit-of-the-am-tree, natron, setseft-seeds, bone-of-the-swordfish, cooked, redfish, cooked, skull-of-crayfish, cooked, honey, and abra-ointment.and 60 Some of the recommended treatments made use of cannabis and incense.Egyptian medicinal use of plants in antiquity is known to be extensive, with some 160 distinct plant products... Amidst the many plant extracts and fruits, the Egyptians also used animal feces and even some metals as treatments. These prescriptions of antiquity were measured out by volume, not weight, which makes their prescription making craft more like cooking than what Pharmacists do today.While their treatments and herbal remedies seem almost boundless, they still included incantations along with some therapeutic remedies.

Medical knowledge in ancient Egypt had an excellent reputation; while rulers of other empires would ask the Egyptian pharaoh to send them their best physician to treat their loved ones.[citation needed] Egyptians had some knowledge of human anatomy. For example, in the classic mummification process, mummifiers knew how to insert a long hooked implement through a nostril, breaking the thin bone of the braincase and removing the brain. They also had a general idea that inner organs are in the body cavity. They removed the organs through a small incision in the left groin. Whether this knowledge was passed down to the practitioners is unknown; yet it did not seem to have had any impact on their medical theories.

Egyptian physicians were aware of the existence of the pulse and its connection to the heart. The author of the Smith Papyrus even had a vague idea of the cardiac system. Although he did not know about blood circulation and deemed it unimportant to distinguish between blood vessels, tendons, and nerves. They developed their theory of "channels" that carried air, water, and blood to the body by analogies with the River Nile; if it became blocked, crops became unhealthy. They applied this principle to the body: If a person was unwell, they would use laxatives to unblock the "channels".

The oldest written text mentioning enemas is the Ebers Papyrus and many medications were administered using enemas. One of the many types of medical specialists was an Iri, the Shepherd of the Anus.

Many of their medical practices were effective, such as the surgical procedures given in the Edwin Smith papyrus. Mostly, the physicians' advice for staying healthy was to wash and shave the body, including under the arms, to prevent infections. They also advised patients to look after their diet, and avoid foods such as raw fish or other animals considered to be unclean.

PREFACE

this is the final honest translation from the original papyrus , it took more than seven years to finish , moving from diffrent resources , original scripts , and liberaries .

the hardest problem for me is to recognising the substances names , eventhough it is confusing but in the end it is all about certain substances were used again and again .

maybe the diagnosis was not so clear because the symptoms were just mentioned in one line but now we have the knowledge about the substances connected with the eye treatment , therefore we can use these substances and make them part of our daily consumption .

we always trust the natural resources and this is the point .

PROLOGUE

Egyptian medical papyri are ancient Egyptian texts written on papyrus which permit a glimpse at medical procedures and practices in ancient Egypt. The papyri give details on disease, diagnosis, and remedies of disease, which include herbal remedies, surgery, and magical spells. It is thought there were more medical papyri, but many have been lost due to grave robbing. The largest study of the medical papyri to date has been undertaken by Berlin University and was titled Medizin der alten Ägypter ("Medicine of ancient Egypt").

Early Egyptian medicine was based mostly on a mixture of magic and religious spells. Most commonly "cured" by use of amulets or magical spells, the illnesses were thought to be caused by spiteful behavior or actions. Afterwards, doctors performed various medical treatments if necessary. The instructions for these medical rituals were later inscribed on papyrus scrolls by the priests performing the actions.

Main medical papyri:

Kahun Papyrus
Dated to circa 1800 BCE, the Kahun Gynaecological Papyrus is the oldest known medical text in Egypt. It was found at El-Lahun by Flinders Petrie in 1889, first translated by F. Ll. Griffith in 1893, and published in The Petrie Papyri: Hieratic Papyri from Kahun and Gurob. The papyrus contains 35 separate paragraphs relating to women's health, such as gynaecological diseases, fertility, pregnancy, and contraception. It does not describe surgery.

Ramesseum Papyri :
The Ramesseum medical papyri consist of 17 individual papyri that were found in the great temple of the Ramesseum. They concentrate on the eyes, gynecology, paediatrics, muscles and tendons.

Edwin Smith Papyrus :
Dated to circa 1600 BCE, the Edwin Smith Papyrus is the only surviving copy of part of an ancient Egyptian textbook on trauma surgery. The papyrus takes its name from the Egyptian archaeologist Edwin Smith, who purchased it in the 1860s. The most detailed and sophisticated of the extant medical papyri, it is also the world's oldest surgical text. Written in the hieratic script of the ancient Egyptian language, it is thought to be based on material from a thousand years earlier.The document consists of 22 pages (17 pages on the recto, and 5 pages on the verso). 48 cases of trauma are examined, each with a description of the physical examination, diagnosis, treatment, and prognosis.An important aspect of the text is that it shows that the heart, liver, spleen, kidneys, ureters, and bladder were all known to the Egyptians, along with the fact that the blood vessels were connected to the heart. The entire translation is available online.

Ebers Papyrus
The Ebers Papyrus was also purchased by Edwin Smith in 1862. It takes its name from Georg Ebers who purchased the papyrus in 1872. The papyrus dates to around 1550BC and covers 110 pages, making it the lengthiest of the medical papyri. The papyrus covers many different topics including; dermatology, digestive diseases, traumatic diseases, dentistry and gynecological conditions. It makes many references to treating ailments with spells or religious techniques.[citation needed] One of the most important findings of this papyrus are the references to migraines which shows the condition dates back to this time.

Hearst Papyrus

The Hearst Papyrus was offered in 1901 to the Hearst Expedition in Egypt. It is dated around 2000 BC, though doubts subsist about its authenticity. It concentrated on treatments for problems dealing with the urinary system, blood, hair, and bites. It has been extensively studied since its publication in 1905.

London Papyrus:
The London Medical Papyrus is located in the British Museum and dates back to Tutankhamun. Although in poor condition, study of it has found it to focus on magical spells as remedy for disease.

Berlin Papyrus:
The Greater Berlin Papyrus, also known as the Brugsch Papyrus (Pap. Berl. 3038) was discovered by Giuseppe Passalacqua. It consists of 24 pages and is very similar to the Ebers Papyrus. Later sold to Friedrich Wilhelm IV of Prussia with other objects in 1827 for the Berlin Museum, the Greater Berlin Papyrus was translated into German in 1909.

Carlsberg Papyrus
The Carlsberg Papyrus is the property of the Carlsberg Foundation. The papyrus covers diseases of the eye and pregnancy.

Chester Beatty Medical Papyrus:
The Chester Beatty Medical Papyrus is named after Sir Alfred Chester Beatty who donated 19 papyri to the British Museum. The remedies in these texts are generally related to magic and focus on conditions that involve headaches and anorectal ailments.

Brooklyn Papyrus:
The Brooklyn Papyrus – Focusing mainly on snakebites, the Brooklyn Papyrus speaks of remedial methods for poisons obtained from snakes, scorpions, and tarantulas. The Brooklyn Papyrus currently resides in the Brooklyn Museum

INCANTATIONS

magic spells

A Treatment To Be Applied To The Eyes: Spell:

This is the eye of Horus

Founded by the deities of Ain Shams

And the worshipped (Thoth) brought it from the Ashmonites and from the large courtyard in Ain Shams

And from city (Be) and from city (Deb)

It is said to it: Come, the luxurious eye of Horus

O Eye of Horus, I will come to ward off the divine pain and severe headache which is deadly killing, which is hatefully antagonize , and which hurts ..

My eyes are under my fingers

Save after me ... save ... come ... save '

This spell is said four times when this treatment is taken

Another Spell For The Right Eye:

Do to remove irritation:

...... Like a strenuous flame .. I know your name .. "the gentle " ... I know your name. Tie the right eye with a rag so that it is not difficult or tight on it.

24. Another Spell For The Paralyzed Eyes :

"O mortal death

Which paralyzed the eyes

And made in my eyes this rheum

Do not do the paralysis, nor the rheum , nor the squint ...

Because Anubis ..

Found in fatal death a lot ..

Osiris is eating ..

This night ..

I told you not to see ..

Make yourself in front of me because thot is beside me ..

And they see your name so be wherever I look."

This spell is said four times on Anubis. And on the eye drawn above the cover, and serve beer to it.

Or take and anoint his eye with his hand that is under the sick area, for it will see immediately.

Another treatment:

Bull intestines :Made on fire with wheat and barley (barabi.)

Another Spell:

"O cold cold

Osiris has pain in his nose.

Do not infect him and do not rise to his arm.

turn away.

Isis said:

Let me preserve the parts in it from the things that arise from my son.

Atum said:

"prevent any blindness from him

And push away from him this eye paralysis

That exist in his organ

And your blindness,

And paralysis of my son horus face. "

Isis said:

I'll make my braid which is in him.

So He protects himself by his magic ... I do not make ...

My son (Horis) ...

I gave you in a city (naerit)

I gave you in town (Dennett).

I gave you in a city (kesret)

And I gave you in (Alaeaba) city

And I gave you this in the city of Armant. "

This spell is said and written in ply (paper) and makes seven knots ..

And each one of them is placed in the fire and its water is squeezed and drip into the eyes, and one of them is placed on the surface of the right eye and the other on the surface of the left eye. And one of them is placed in ....

This is said four times.

REMEDY

*The eye diseases and treatment
as mentioned in papyri*

Ebers papyrus:

336. Starting of the Book of Eyes:

Useful Medicines For Tingling Blood In The Eye:

Natron (from upper Egypt) : 1

Honey : 1

Whetstone (stone type) :1

Treatment Of Watery Eye I.e: Tearing

Frankincense : 1

Myrrh : 1

Sumac : 1

Lead rust : 1

A Remedy To Heal Eye Irritation :

note from author : maybe this condition is episcleritis , feeling of something hurt the eye .

Natron salt : 1

Lead oxide : 1

Patina : 1

Honey : 1

After that, make a compound ointment for it :

Spring wax : 1

Copper sulfate : 1

Frankincense : 1

Lead rust : 1

And piece of rotten wood : 1

And frankincense : 1

And 1 goose fat

And lead rust from the land of <u>Aqar</u> (desert land) <u>:</u> 1

And Antimony : 1

And 1 oil

It is placed by a period of four days

And there is no great danger

337- Another Treatment To Strengthen Eyesight:

First day : Lake water : 1

The second day : honey: 1 and antimony: 1

They are placed for one day

If the blood remains in it, then put honey : 1

And antimony : 1

They are placed on it for two days.

And if water (i.e. tears) comes out of it a lot, then do for it a remedy for rot (i.e. corruption), which is:

Seeds of plant called <u>aw</u> : 1

<u>Genzar</u> (patina : copper rust) fillings : 1

Frankincense : 1

Ranunculus (Buttercup) hair : 1

To be cooked and placed on it.

338- ....(Unclear Text)

Acacia leaf 1

Antimony : 1

Patina : 1

Colocynth : 1

Water : 1

Dish and put it at sleep time .

339- Others To Remove The Darkness Of The Eye:

Myrrh : 1

Siwar " Musk" : 1

marble powder (calcium carbonate)

Coloynth : 1

Sea cyperus : 1

Patina : 1

Deer shit : 1

Shit of Qiddiya (a kind of huge goat) 1

White oil

-Put it in water, stay in the dew, filter, and apply it for four days.

There Is Another Saying :

brush an Eyeliner to it with Feather of an eagle bird.

Other Treatment:

Copper vitriol (copper sulphate) : 1

Yarrows : 1

The roots of papyrus : 1

And after that I make wax crumbs for it

And put it on the back of the eye.

341- Other:

To remove eye pain:

Antimony : 1

<u>Midad</u> : *has this meaning : a color used to write: i.e : ink 1

Eyeliner

342- Other: For Eye Hernia:

Put it at bedtime on the back of the eyes

Seed of <u>zend</u> ? : 1

The heart of carthamus : 1

Antimony : 1

Water : 1

grind smooth and mix together and put on the back of the eyes.

Another Treatment :

Colocynth : 1

<u>Pulb of (AZIT)</u> : 1

Add oil : 1

And cereals are made and dried and grinded after being dried, and placed on the back of the eyes.

344- Other:

Made from:

Antimony : 1

Colocynth : 1

Lead rust : 1

Crocodile shit : 1

Musk : 1

Red natron : 1

Honey : 1

Mix one thing and put it on the back of the eyes.

345- Other: For Retraction Of The Pupil (I.e. Atrophy):

Ebony fillings 1

Natron from upper Egypt: 1

It is mixed with water and placed on the eyes a lot.

346 - Other: For Removal Of Pale (I.e. Pain) Eyes:

Antimony : 1

Lead oxide (red lead) : 1

Lead rust : 1

Red natron 1

Put it on the back of the eyes.

347 - To Remove The White Of The Eye (Corneal Opacity):

Turtle glands (hawksbill sea turtle) : 1

Honey : 1

It is placed on the back of the eyes.

348 - Other: To Remove Congestion In The Eyes:

Midad (color used to write) : 1

Patina : 4

Antimony : 1

Dror (rotten wood) : 1

Colocynth : 1

Water : 1

Grind fine and place on the eye.

349 - Another Drug That Works For The Point Or Cloud That Is Held In The Eye:

Dry baby feces : 1

And honey : 1

They are made in dough and placed on the back of the eyes.

350 - Other: For Removal Of Pain Of Eyes:

hawksbill sea turtle glands : 1

And fragrance : 1

They are placed over the eyes.

351 - Other: For Burning Of The Eyes :

The roasted ox liver in the fire

 is placed on it, it is tested.

352 - Other: For Removing Congestion In The Eyes (And Originally Removing Blood From The Eyes):

Frankincense : 1

Turmeric : 1

They are placed on the eyes

353 - Other: To Prevent Tangle (Strangulation) From Sore Eyes:

Colocynth : 1

Antimony : 1

Tree throne : <u>zind</u> : arbre a epine.

It is placed on the back of the eyes.

354 : Other: For Fatting Of Eyes :

(Perhaps what is called pterygium by the public)

Antimony : 1

Patina : 1

Lead oxide :1

musk : 1

Honey 1

-Put on the back of the eyes.

355- Other: To Remove Papules From The Eyes: (Trachoma):

Antimony : 1

Patina : 1

Colocynth : 1

Dror (rotten wood)

Copper vitriol

Mix with water and put on the back of the eyes.

356 - Others: For The Blindness Of The Eyes (I.e. For The Blind):

It is taken from the eyes of pig the water that is in them

Real antimony : 1

Lead oxide : 1

Honey : 1

It is made fine, mixes one thing, and injected into a person's ear, and he gets cured immediately

Take a closer look, it is tried, and recite the following magic spell :

"I brought this to be placed in this store to ward off harm (and originally to push harm)"

357 - Other: To Remove The Blindness Of The Eye From The Pupil:

Dry myrrh .

It is served in sour dough and placed on the back of the eyes.

358- Other:

Colocynth

Mixed with honey and placed on the back of the eyes.

359 - To Treat Eyesight:

Antimony : 1

Midad (color used in writing) : 1

Colocynth : 1

Copper sulfate : 1

Antimony (male?) : 1

Make one thing and put it in the eyes.

360 - Others To Remove The Linen From The Eyes (Begin With A Spell):

" There is sound in the southbound sky

During the night.

And there is a rampage in the northbound sky.

The column has fallen into the water.

And hit the sailors of the sun with their oars

Their Heads fell into the water.

Who came near - the column – he will find it.

I brought it ..

I found it ..

I drew your heads

And raised your necks

I come back where what was cut from you.

I brought you to push the deadly divine ailments with death..:

Open the mouth and say to the hawksbill sea turtle glands mixed with honey to be placed on the back of the eyes.

361 - Other: To Eliminate Sore Eyes:

Maidenhair fern

Myrrh from Byblos (a city in Phenicia called Jbeil: gebeil)

They are made soft in the water and the person bandages the back of his eyes to heal.

362- Other:

Grease from a donkey's jaw

It is mixed in cold water that a person puts on his temple and he heals immediately.

363- Other: To Heal The Temples:

Turmeric in cold water

The person places it on his temple and heals instantly.

364 - Other:

Tooth of a donkey

To be grinded in water and a person puts it on his temple and heals.

365- Other: To Remove The Tumor From The Eye Called (Addt):

Ebers said it is case of pterygion, meaning the back, and Joachim the German agreed with him and Louring said that it is a wound. Hirschberg said in his book on Explaining the Eyes, Folio 49, that it is eye cancer.

Shit of bird called the Egyptian (Hanut) : 1

lake salt : 1

frankincense : 1

mix together and placed inside the eye.

366 -To Remove Inflammation From The Eye:

Natron Saidi (from upper Egypt) : placed in boza water

To be placed in the eye and heal it.

367 - Others: To Remove The Blockage In The Gills: (Perhaps They Are Tear Ducts That Connect To The Eye):

Antimony 1/32

Whetstone : 1/16

hdm (incense type)

midad 1 \ 64

green myrrh 1/64

Natron Saidi (from upper Egypt) : 1/64

They are grinded fine, mixed together and placed in the eye, and you will be cured immediately.

368 - Other: To Remove The White Of The Eye:

Real antimony , placed in a hen of water for four days, with replenishment of water.

Then it is placed in goose fat for four days

Then it is moistened with the milk of a woman who gave birth to a male and dried for nine days.

Then it is sauced and placed on it a grain of myrrh.

And eyeliner it to those whose eyes are white.

369 – Addt :

See 365

1 - After incantation: put sour honey or honeycomb on it for four days

2 - copper sulfate 1/8

Antimony : 1/8

Dror (rotten wood): 1 \ 8

Natron from upper egypt : 1 \ 8

Grind to one thing and put it on it for four days.

370 - Other:

Agamas shit : 1

Natron (from upper Egypt) :1

Antimony : 1

Honey : 1

Grind to one thing and put it on the eyes.

• Durar(dror) is the rotten wood and is still used to heal circumcision.

371 - Other:

Lead oxide : 1

Antimony : 1

Sour honey : 1

One thing is stunned and placed on the eyes.

372 - Other :

Copper sulfate : 1

Honey : 1

It is put on the eyes for four days

373- Other :

Lead oxide : 1

Antimony : 1

Sour honey : 1

Made one thing and put on the eyes .

374 - Other:

Lead oxide : 1

Dror (rotten wood) : 1

(door) Qusi (a type of stone from Qus, a village in Upper Egypt) 1

Copper sulfate 1

Ostrich egg 1

Natron (from upper Egypt) : 1

Column sulfur powder 1

Honey 1

Make one thing and put it on the eyes.

375 - Other:

Black whetstone : 1

Frankincense : 1

Antimony : 1

Honey 1

It is placed on it for a period of four days.

376 - Other (Beneficial) Secretion Of The Eye (Perhaps Conjunctivitis)

Scavengers 5

Of statue 1 *

Castor paper (or scrap) 1

Honey 1

Dish finely and mix and put on

* What falls from a statue - sculpting the statue - when it was made.

377 - Other: For Eye Hernia:

Antimony : 1/8

Doum (Hyphaene thebaica) 1 \ 4

Whetstone 1/4

Ink : 1/64

Natron from upper Egypt 1/64

Myrrh 1/64

Mix it together and put it on the eye.

378 - Other: To Remove The Rise Of Water To The Eyes: Glucoma

(I.e., blue water scientifically known as a glucoma)

Note from author : it was mentioned in the last translation as cataract but cataract is white water so I edited it to glaucoma which is blue water just for the honesty of translation I had to clarify that .

Real lapis lazuli : 1

Clay : 1

Sinan (whetstone): 1

Milk :1

Antimony : 1

Nile alluvium

Mastic

Dill

Mix together and put on the back of the eyes.

379 - Other:

Sehtet : 1

goose fat : 1

Honey : 1

Mix it together and put it on the eye for four days.

380 - Other:

Copper sulfate 1

Clay (adhesive clay for pottery) 1

A substance called (Berhadov) 1

Grind and mix together and encompasses the eye.

381 - Other: To Ward Off The Point From The Eye:

Note from author : this may be cataract .

Myrrh 1

Colocynth (start to be yellow) 1

Honey 1

It is made fine, and kept in a rag and placed on the eye that has the point.

382 - To Ward Off White In The Eye:

Granite stone

Dish fine, sift with rag, and put(i.e. keep) on the eye.

383 - To Prevent Strabismus From The Eyes:

Acacia leaf1

Colocynth powder 1

Granite stone 1

It is dished and placed on the eye (and originally eyes are placed on it)

384 - To Ward Off Blood From The Eyes:

Two Pottery bowels :

One containing Doum powder and the milk of a woman who gave birth to a male

And the other has milk

Keep to stay overnight

In the morning the eyes are filled from this doum, and after that the eyes are washed with this milk 4 times (every day).

385 - To Ward Off The Rise Of Water In The Eye:

Come, O clay
Come, O Blessed clay .

Violated things are in Horis eye .

Come on, vomit

To the eye of idol Atum

Come on, Intractable diseases

Emerging from the eye of osiris.

It came and turned off the water

And pus, blood and around the eyes

And rheum and blindness and tears

From the eye of the idol

The deadly pain is death, and tingling , and everything is bad

That exist in these eyes:

To open the mouth.

It is said three times on the clay , and it is mixed with honey and placed in wine and mixed with Cyperus(nutsedges) and is used according to the rules.

386 - Other Things To Eyeliner The Sore Eyes:

Henna heads

Colocynth (Handhal)

honey

goose fat

(Equivalent quantities)

It is placed on the back of the eye, it is really useful a hundred thousand times.

387 - Other: To Soften The Blood Vessels In The Eye:

Dry myrrh

Milk cream

Clay

Iron filings

(Equivalent quantities)

It is placed on the back of the eye.

388- Treatment During The Winter To The Winter Months:

Antimony

 Natron grains

Ink

Copper sulfate

Rotten wood

(Equivalent quantities)

Placed on the eye.

389 - Other: Eyeliner For The Eyes In Summer, Winter And Flood Season:

Antimony

Clay

Lapis lazuli

honey

Lead rust

(Equivalent quantities)

It is made as tablets and is placed on the eye.

391 - Al-Khenan: Cold : Sinusitis

To ward off sinusitis (a disease of the head and eye)

Antimony 1

Rotten wood 1/8

Sinan (whetstone) 1/16

Copper sulfate 1/16

Midad(ink) 1 \ 64

Dry myrrh 1/64

392 Treating The Eye And Everything Harmful That Happens In It:

brain

divided to two halves , making half of it on honey with which the eye can be applied at night, the other half of which is dried, and it shall be grinded soft, and applied with it in the morning.

393 - To Strengthen Eyesight:

It is used in the first month of winter to the second of winter:

Male antimony

Antimony

Sinan (whetstone)

(Equivalent quantities)

Placed on the eye.

394- Other:

Natron (from upper Egypt)

Antimony

(Equivalent quantities)

It is placed on the eye.

395- Other:

Colcynth

Antimony 1

Honey 1

It is placed on the eyes in equal amounts.

396 - Other For Eye Hernia:

A new bowl piece from clay covered with dough was placed over the eye over and over

397 - Other For Eye Hernia:

Antimony

beef(cow meat)

It is placed on the eye.

398 - Other For Eye Hernia:

Antimony 3

Honey 3

It is placed on the eye.

399 - Other For Eye Hernia:

Antimony

Colocynth fresh water

Sour Honey .

It is placed on the eyes.

400 – Other Treatment An Eyeliner:

Antimony 2

Honey 4

Clay 1/4

Lead rust 1/4

Real lapis lazuli

grind and put in the eye.

401- Another Solution:

Antimony 2

Goose Fat 2

Water 4

Drip into the eye.

402- To Remove The White Layer From The Eye:

Antimony

Rotten wood

Grind soft and put on the eyes.

403 - Others:

Midad (ink) 1

Antimony 1

Water

Grind soft and put on the eyes.

404 - Other:

ebony

antimony

Water

Grind soft and put on the eyes.

405- Others:

Bagrus gallbladder (fish)

Antimony

Grind soft and put on the eyes.

406 - Other:

Milk cream

Milk

Mix soft and put on the eyes.

407 - Other: To Remove The Blood From Eyes :

Antimony : 1

Lead oxide : 1

Lead rust : 1

Red natron : 1

Grind and put on the back of the eyes.

408 - Others: To Remove The Red Dust From The Eyes (I.e. Their Opacity)

Colocynth

Acacia paper

The milk of a woman gave birth to a male

Mix together and put on the back of the eye.

409 – Aadt (I.e. Harm)

Antimony 1/2

Ostrich egg 3/4

They are mixed soft and placed on the back of the eye.

410 - Other:

Antimony : 2

Honey : 1/64

Lead rust : 1/16

Lead oxide 1/8

Sinan (whetstone) 1/8

Grind soft and put on the back of the eye.

411- Other:

Lead oxide 1/32

Lead rust 1/4

Antimony 1/32

Sinan (whetstone) 1/16

Honey 2 ¼

Grind soft and put on the eye

412- Others:

Black Watis (stone type used to grill in) 1/32

Frankincense 1 \ 8

Clay 1

Honey 1

It is bandage it to the eye (and the origin is its face it to the eye)

413 – Aadt :

Lead oxide 1/64

Lead rust 1/64

Sour honey 1/8

Antimony : 1/8

Sinan (whetstone) 1/32

It is grinded fine and placed on the back of the eye.

414 – Other: For Eye Hernia:

Milk cream

Milk of a woman who gave birth to a male.

They are mixed together and drip into the eye.

415- To Remove Alopecia, Which Means The Loss Of Hair, Clouding, Pain And Headache In The Eyes:

Note from author : this is A dermatological condition maybe ophiasis :

Rotten wood : 1

Clay :1

Colocynth powder 1

Acacia leaf 1

Ebony fillings 1

<u>KABB</u> extract (i.e., acid) 1

Mix together and make dry bread and mix with water, then apply on the eyes.

416 – Blennorrhoea (Conjunctivitis):

Clay 2

Ink 1

Antimony 2 1/2 (2.5)

Natron : 1

Lead rust : 1/8

Mix with water and put on the back of the eyes.

417 - Other: Blennorrhoea:

Lead oxide : 1

Goose fat : 1

Paint the back of the eye with it and see well, it is real.

418 - To Remove A Cold In The Nose:

Antimony : 1

Rotten wood : 1

Dry myrrh : 1

Honey : 1

- It will be painted as eyeliner with it for four days, then look well, it is real.

419 - Other: Kohl Made By The Priest (Khoy):

Antimony : 1

Clay : 1

Natron from southbound : 1

Natron from northbound : 1

Lead oxide : 1

Rotten wood : 1

Sour honey : 1.

420- For Removing Blindness From The Eyes:

Colocynth

Grind it finely, sift it with a rag, mix it with honey and place it in the eyes.

421- To Ward Off Pain From The Organs Of The Eye:

Clay

Frankincense

Lead oxide

It is grinded and placed on the eye.

422 - Other: Eye Treatment, Said By An Asian From The City Of Byblos, Which Is Jubail:

Honey 1

Dates 1

Fresh dates 1

Barley 1

Tragacanth : 1

Lead oxide : 1

Solvent of khadla : 1? (note from the author : khadla has two meaning : small grape and euphorbia ammak)

Salt 1

Acacia asak : 1

Antimony : 1

fat

fresh oil .

- prepared as a remedy.

423: To Remove Conjunctivitis From The Eye:

Antimony : 1

Sinan(whetstone) : 1

Rotten wood : 1

Apply it to the eye(paint)

424 - To Remove Hair From The Eye:

Myrrh :1

The blood of the agamas 1

Bat blood 1

For hair removal (ie, to prevent germination of hair)is placed on it until it heals.

425 - Other: To Prevent Hair Growth In The Eye After Removing It:

Frankincense , grinded with agamas shit 1

And the blood of a bull 1

And donkey blood 1

Pig blood 1

And dog blood 1

Deer blood 1

Then antimony : 1

And clay 1

- It is made soft and mixed with this blood, and replaced with this hair after removing it, so it does not sprout.

426 - Other:

Bat blood : 1

A piece of clay bowl : 1

Honey 1

- They are grinded finely and put on this hair after removing it.

427 - Other:

Cow fat 1

faq (cooked oil) 1

hemaaa afnit ! (mud in which this worm grows) 1

They are mixed together and placed in place of this hair after removing it.

428 - Other:

Bird's gland (wat) – and arundo 1

It is grinded in it and place it in the place of this hair after removing it.

429 - To Prevent Hair Germination In The Eye After Removing It:

Hornet shit : 1 (note from author : sometime it's meant by honey)

Lead oxide : 1

Urine : 1

It is mixed and applied to replace this hair after removing it.

430 - To Remove Pimples (I.e., Trachoma) From The Eye:

Sinan (whetStone) 1

Antimony : 1

Rotten wood : 1

The eyes are covered with it.

431 - To Remove Fat From The Eye:

Stone carver <u>(doos?)</u> "note from the author : it's a stone for polishing swords"

It is mixed with dough and placed frequently.

751 - To Remove The Nso(Discomfort With The Eye):

Nutmeg : 1

<u>Auf</u> (a good smelling plant) 1

<u>Zeiss</u> (vegetable) 1

Papyrus 1

Fresh beer 1/3

- It is filtered, and the person with nso eats it.

INDEX

substances

Acacia asak /
Acacia leaf (paper) ////
Agamas (shit / /) (blood /)
Antimony
///
Antimony male //
Baby shit /
Bagrus (gallbladder) /
Barley /
Bat blood //
Beef /
Beer /
Boza /
Brain /
Bull intestine /
Bull liver /
Bull blood /
Carthamus /
Castor paper /
Clay //////////////
Colocynth ////////////////
Copper sulfate /////////
Copper vitriol /
Cow fat /
Crocodile shit /
Cyperus (nutsedges) /
Dates //
Deer shit /
Deer blood /
Dill /
Dog blood /
Donkey jaw /
Donkey tooth /
Donkey blood /
Doum (Hyphaene thebaica) //

Eagle feather /
Ebony fillings ///
Fat /
Fir
Fragrance /
Frankincense . //////////
Goat shit /
Goose fat /////
Granite //
hawksbill sea turtle (glands) ///
henna /
Honey ////////////////////////////
Ink /////////
Iron filllings /
Lake salt /
Lake water /
lapis lazuli //
Lead oxide ///////////////
Lead rust ///////////
Maidenhair fern /
Marble (brushed or powder) /
Mastic /
Milk //
Milk cream ///
Milk of woman who gave birth to male ////
Musk ///
Myrrh ///////////
Natron from upper Egypt ////////
Natron salt //////
Nile alluvium /
Nutmeg /
Oil ////
Ostrich egg //
Papyrus /
Papyrus roots /
Patina //////

pig eyes /
pig blood /
Ranunculus (Buttercup)
Red lapis lazuli /
Red natron ///
Rotten wood ////////////
Salt /
Scavengers /
Sea cyperus /
Sour honey /////
Sulfer powder /
 Sumac /
Tragacanth /
Tree throne /
Turmeric //
Urine /
Water //////////
Wax //
Whetstone //////////
Whetstone black /
White oil /
Yarrows /

REFRENCES

References
1.WEKIPEDIA
2. ^ Jouanna, Jacques; Allies, Neil (2012), "Egyptian Medicine and Greek Medicine", Greek Medicine from Hippocrates to Galen, Brill, pp. 3–20, JSTOR 10.1163/j.ctt1w76vxr.6
3. ^ Said, Galal Zaki (17 November 2013). "Orthopaedics in the dawn of civilisation, practices in ancient Egypt". International Orthopaedics. 38 (4): 905–909. doi:10.1007/s00264-013-2183-z. ISSN 0341-2695. PMC 3971265. PMID 24240438.
4. ^ "Edwin Smith papyrus (Egyptian medical book)". Encyclopedia Britannica (Online ed.). Retrieved 1 January 2016.
5. ^ Arab, Sameh M. "Medicine in Ancient Egypt – Part 1". Arab World Books. Retrieved 18 November 2011.
6. ^ Fagan, Brian M. (2004). The Seventy Great Inventions of the Ancient World. Thames & Hudson. ISBN 978-0-50005130-6.
7. ^ WEINBERGER, B. (1946). FURTHER EVIDENCE THAT DENTISTRY WAS PRACTICED IN ANCIENT EGYPT, PHOENICIA AND GREECE. Bulletin of the History of Medicine,20(2), 188–195. Retrieved from http://www.jstor.org/stable/44441040
8. ^ Jump up to:a b DAWSON, W. (1927). THE BEGINNINGS OF MEDICINE: MEDICINE AND SURGERY IN ANCIENT EGYPT. Science Progress in the Twentieth Century (1919–1933), 22(86), 275–284. Retrieved from http://www.jstor.org/stable/43430010
9. ^ Griffith, F. Ll. (1898). The Petrie Papyri: Hieratic Papyri from Kahun and Gurob. London: Bernard Quaritch. (Please note the book pages run from back to front.)
10. ^ Bynum, W. F.; Hardy, Anne; Jacyna, Stephen; Lawrence, Christopher; Tansey, E.M. (2006). "The Rise of Science in Medicine, 1850–1913". The Western Medical Tradition: 1800–2000. Cambridge University Press. pp. 198–199. ISBN 978-0-521-47565-5.
11. ^ Dollinger, André. "The Kahun Gynaecological Papyrus". An introduction to the history and culture of Pharaonic Egypt. Kibbutz Reshafim. Retrieved 21 April 2012.
12. ^ Jump up to:a b c d e Dollinger, André (December 2002). "Ancient Egyptian Medicine". An introduction to the history and

culture of Pharaonic Egypt. Kibbutz Reshafim.

13.   ^ Jump up to:a b Breasted, James Henry (1930). The Edwin Smith Papyrus. Chicago, Illinois: The University of Chicago Press.

14.   ^ Allen, James P (2005). The Art of Medicine in Ancient Egypt. New York: The Metropolitan Museum of Art. ISBN 978-0-300-10728-9.

15.   ^ Jump up to:a b Bryan, Cyril (1932). The Ebers Papyrus. New York: D. Appleton and Company.

16.   ^ Jump up to:a b c d Nunn, John F. (1996). Ancient Egyptian Medicine. Transactions of the Medical Society of London. 113. Norman, Oklahoma: University of Oklahoma Press. pp. 57–68. ISBN 978-0-8061-2831-3. PMID 10326089.

17.   ^ Ritner, Robert K. (April 2000). "Innovations and Adaptations in Ancient Egyptian Medicine". Journal of Near Eastern Studies. 59(2): 107–117. doi:10.1086/468799. JSTOR 545610. PMID 16468204. S2CID 39263523.

18.   ^ Dollinger, André. "Herbal Medicine". An introduction to the history and culture of Pharaonic Egypt. Kibbutz Reshafim. Retrieved 9 October 2015.

19.   ^ Parkins, Michael D.; Szekrenyes, J. (March 2001). "Pharmacological Practices of Ancient Egypt" (PDF). Proceedings of the 10th Annual History of Medicine Days. Calgary, Alberta, Canada: The University of Calgary. pp. 5–11.

20.   ^ "What progress did the Egyptians make in medical knowledge?". Medicine Through Time: Model Questions and Answers. Passmores Academy. Archived from the original on 1 May 2008. Retrieved 1 January 2016.

21.   ^ Magner, Lois (1992). A History of Medicine. Boca Raton, Florida: CRC Press. p. 31. ISBN 978-0-8247-8673-1.

22.   ^ Stiefel, Marc; Shaner, Arlene; Schaefer, Steven D. (February 2006). "The Edwin Smith Papyrus: The Birth of Analytical Thinking in Medicine and Otolaryngology". The Laryngoscope. 116 (2): 182–188. doi:10.1097/01.mlg.0000191461.08542.a3. ISSN 0023-852X. PMID 16467701. S2CID 35256503.

23.   ^ El-Aref, Nevine (December 2006). "Too big for a coffin". Al-Ahram Weekly. Cairo, Egypt: Al-Ahram. Archived from the origin-

alon 18 November 2014. Retrieved 1 January 2016.

24.   ^ Hawass, Zahi (2003). "The tomb of the physician Qar". Hidden Treasures of the Egyptian Museum: One Hundred Masterpieces from the Centennial Exhibition (Supreme Council of Antiquities ed.). Cairo, Egypt: American University in Cairo Press. p. xx. ISBN 978-977424778-1.

25.   ^ Lauer, Jean Philippe (3 January 2013). "Imhoteb Museum". Egypt Tourism News. Egypt Tourism Board. Retrieved 1 January2016.

26.   ^ Jackson, Russell (6 December 2006). "Mummy of ancient doctor comes to light". The Scotsman. Edinburgh. Retrieved 24 March2011.

27.   ^ Greiner, Ryan (2001). "Ancient Egyptian Medicine". Creighton University Virtual Museums. Creighton University. Retrieved 2 April 2011.

28.   ^ Herodotus (25 February 2006) [First published 1890]. An Account of Egypt (from The History of Herodotus Translated into English, Vol. I, Pages 115–208). Translated by Macaulay, G. C. Project Gutenberg.

29.   ^ Jump up to:a b Arab, Sameh M. "Medicine in Ancient Egypt – Part 3". Arab World Books. Retrieved 18 November 2011.

30.   ^ "Medicine in Ancient Egypt", SpringerReference, Springer-Verlag, 2011, doi:10.1007/springerreference_78530

31.   ^ Gordan, Andrew H.; Shwabe, Calvin W. (2004). The Quick and the Dead: Biomedical Theory in Ancient Egypt. Egyptological Memoirs. Leiden: Brill Academic Publishers. p. 154. ISBN 978-90-04-12391-5.

32.   ^ Grajetzki, Wolfram; Quirke, Stephen (2003). "Knowledge and production: the House of Life". Digital Egypt for Universities. University College London. Retrieved 18 November 2011.

33.   ^ Bareš, Ladislav (2005). "The Shaft Tomb of Udjahorresnet". Czech Institute of Egyptology. Charles University in Prague. Retrieved 1 January 2016.

34.   ^ Wood, Gemma Ellen (4 July 2012). "Dispelling the myth – Herodotus, Cambyses, and Egyptian religion #1". The Egyptiana Emporium. Retrieved 1 January 2016.

35.   ^ Jump up to:a b c Agut-Labordère, Damien (2013). "The Saite Period: The Emergence of a Mediterranean Power". Ancient Egyptian Administration. Handbook of Oriental Studies. Leiden: Brill Academic Publishers. pp. 965–1027. ISBN 978-90-04-24952-3.

36.   ^ "Wedjahor-Resne". Livius.org. Jona Lendering. 22 August 2015. Retrieved 1 January 2016.

37.   ^ Fonahn, Adolf (1 January 1909). "Der altägyptische Arzt Iwti". Archiv für Geschichte der Medizin. 2 (5): 375–378. JSTOR 20772830.

38.   ^ Fonahn, Adolf (February 1909). "Der altägyptische Arzt Iwti". Archiv für Geschichte der Medizin (in German). 2 (5): 375–378. JSTOR 20772830

39.   Marry, Austin (January 21, 2004). "Ancient Egyptian Medical Papyri". Ancient Egypt Fan. Eircom Limited. Retrieved 2007-10-24.

40.   ^ "medicine, health and wellbeing". EgyptologyOnline.com. Archived from the original on March 30, 2010. Retrieved 2007-10-26.

41.   ^ Worton, Michael; Wilson-Tagoe, Nana (2004). National Healths: Gender, Sexuality and Health in a Cross-Cultural Context. London: UCL Press/Cavendish Publishing. p. 192. ISBN 978-1-84472-017-0. LCCN 2005295595.

42.   ^ "History of the Library: late Middle Kingdom manuscripts from a tomb under the Ramesseum". Digital Egypt for Universities. University College London. 2003. Retrieved 2007-10-26.

43.   ^ DiPaolo, Anthony C. (November 12, 2009). "The Papyrus Page". Anthony's Egyptology & Archaeology. Osiris Designs. Retrieved 2007-10-24.

44.   ^ Martin, Andrew J. (2005-07-27). "Academy Papyrus to be Exhibited at the Metropolitan Museum of Art" (Press release). The New York Academy of Medicine. Archived from the original on November 27, 2010. Retrieved 2008-08-12.

45.   ^ Wilkins, Robert H. (March 1964). "Neurosurgical Classic-

XVII (Edwin Smith Surgical Papyrus)". Journal of Neurosurgery. 21 (3): 240–244. doi:10.3171/jns.1964.21.3.0240. PMID 14127631. translation of 13 cases from Breasted, James Henry (1930) pertaining to injuries of the skull and spinal cord, with commentary.

46.   ^ "A Brief History of Migraines". Migraine and Headaches. Archived from the original on December 6, 2008. Retrieved 2007-10-24.

47.   ^ Hickey, Todd M.; O'Connell, Elisabeth (2003). "The Hearst Medical Papyrus". The Center for the Tebtunis Papyri). Bancroft Library, University of California, Berkeley. Retrieved 2007-10-25.

48.   ^ Owen, Antoinette; Danzing, Rachel (1993). "The History and Treatment of the Papyrus Collection at The Brooklyn Museum". In Espinosa, Robert (ed.). The Book and Paper Group Annual, Volume 12, 1993. American Institute for Conservation of Historic and Artistic Works. ISSN 0887-8978. LCCN 87640038.

49.   ^ Jump up to:a b Sadek, Ashraf Alexandre (January 2001). "Some Aspects of Medicine in Pharonic Egypt". 50.History of Medicine. Australian Academy of Medicine & Surgery.

 51."RCP". Archived from the original on 2007-09-28. Retrieved 2009-09-05.

52.Sandstead, Harold H.; Wagner, Conrad (2002-06-01). "William J. Darby, 1913–2001". The Journal of Nutrition. 132 (6): 1103–1106. doi:10.1093/jn/132.6.1103. ISSN 0022-3166. PMID 12042417.

53. Alt, Howard L. (1964-06-01). "Blood Diseases". Archives of Internal Medicine. 113 (6): 925. doi:10.1001/archinte.1964.00280120125054. ISSN 0003-9926.

 54."PROFILE". ambassadors.net. Retrieved 2017-10-27.
International Congress of the History of Medicine
Ear, Nose and Throat in Ancient Egypt
55.Paul life
"Biomedical | Library | Vanderbilt University". www.mc.vanderbilt.edu. Retrieved 2017-10-27.
56.Letter from Paul Ghalioungui to C.L. Gemmill

"Naturwissenschaften und Medizin". www.kv5.de. Retrieved 2017-10-27.

57. 2001, Franz-Andre Sondervorst, Chronique de SIHM

58. David, R. (2008). "Redirecting". Lancet. 372 (9652): 1802–3. doi:10.1016/S0140-6736(08)61749-3. PMID 19048654. S2CID 35822210.

59. Dr. Paul Ghalioungui (1982), "The West denies Ibn Al Nafis's contribution to the discovery of the circulation", Symposium on Ibn al-Nafis, Second International Conference on Islamic Medicine: Islamic Medical Organization, Kuwait (cf. The West denies Ibn Al Nafis's contribution to the discovery of the circulation Archived 2009-08-25 at the Wayback Machine, Encyclopedia of Islamic World)

60. Yehia El-Rakhawi interview at Al-Ahram weekly Journal Archived 2009-08-07 at the Wayback Machine

Egyptian Medicine by Carloe Reeves 1992

62. "FindArticles.com | CBSi". findarticles.com. Retrieved 2017-10-27.

IDEO Archived 2011-07-24 at the Wayback Machine

63. "Remy Motte, Antiquaire, spécialiste boiseries et parquets anciens". Archived from the original on 2009-09-03. Retrieved 2009-09-13.

64. IDEO Archived 2011-07-24 at the Wayback Machine

65. "piccione, hist330, course bibliography". spinner.cofc.edu. Retrieved 2017-10-27.

66. Ghalioungui, Paul (1987). The Ebers papyrus: A new English translation, commentaries and glossaries. Academy of Scientific Research and Technology. ASIN B0006ERXEG.

67. "Paul Ghalioungui Books - List of books by Paul Ghalioungui". www.allbookstores.com. Retrieved 2017-10-27.

68. IDEO Archived 2011-07-24 at the Wayback Machine

69. Ghalioungui, Paul (1983). La médecine des pharaons: Magie et science médicale dans l'Egypte ancienne (in French). Paris: R. Laffont. ISBN 9782221011799.

70. Ghalioungui, Paul (1983). The physicians of Pharonic Egypt. Al-Ahram Center for Scientific Translations. ASIN B0006YCXJG.

71 . Ghalioungui, Paul (1983). The physicians of Pharaonic Egypt (First ed.). Mainz a.Rh: Available from the U.S. Dept. of Commerce, National Technical Information Service. ISBN 9783805306003.

72. "Books by National Library of Medicine U S". 2014-02-12. Archived from the original on 2014-02-12.

73. "Journal of the History of Medicine and Allied Sciences | Oxford Academic". OUP Academic. Retrieved 2017-10-27.

74. The Physicians Of Phanasonic Egypt book review by Raja Reddy, B.I.I.H.M.Vol.XIV(1-4) Archived 2009-04-10 at the Wayback Machine

75 ."Islamic Medical Manuscripts : Catalogue - Commentaries 2". www.nlm.nih.gov. Retrieved 2017-10-27.

76 . "Archived copy" (PDF). Archived from the original (PDF) on 2008-12-20. Retrieved 2009-09-06.

77. Ghalioungui, Paul (1979). Kul-- lā ta'kul (in Arabic). Cairo: Dār al-Ma'ārif. ISBN 9789772478088.

78 . IDEO Archived 2011-07-24 at the Wayback Machine

79 . IDEO Archived 2011-07-24 at the Wayback Machine

80 . Food history Ghalioungui, Paul (1973). The house of life;: Per ankh. Magic and medical science in ancient Egypt ([2. herz. druk] ed.). Amsterdam: B. M. Israel. ISBN 9789060780626.

81 . Kinnaer, Jacques. "The Ancient Egypt Site". www.ancient-egypt.org. Retrieved 2017-10-27.

82. ABD AL-LATIF (AL-BAGHDADI) Maqalatann fi-l-Hawass wa Masa'il Tabi'iya, Kuwait, Government Press, 83 . 1972; texte arabe édité par Ghalioungui Paul et Abdou Said Archived 2009-09-05 at the Wayback Machine

84 . Ghalioungui, Paul (1965). Magic and Medical Science in Ancient Egypt (Reprint ed.). Barnes And Noble. ASIN B001TD8ZOU.

85 . Magic and Medical Science in Ancient Egypt Archived 2011-05-18 at the Wayback Machine

86 . "The Oldest Medical Books in the World | Ancient Medicine | World Research Foundation". www.wrf.org. Retrieved 2017-10-27.

87 . "Archived copy". Archived from the original on 2011-07-06.

Retrieved 2009-09-13.

Amazon.com

88 . "AAMS - Australian Academy of Medicine and Surgery". www.aams.org.au. Retrieved 2017-10-27.

89 . Ghalioungui, Paul (1965). Health and healing in ancient Egypt,: A pictorial essay. Dar al-Maaref. ASIN B0006FF400.

BOOKS BY THIS AUTHOR

The Heart: Ancient Egyptian Cardiology

ancient egyptian cardiology is the original prescriptions from different papyri . tracing the substances and breaking the spells and names .
this book is a seed for discoveries in the field of medicine .

The Time: Metaphysical Study

A mystery , which comes before death mystery . and it has been never solved .
Starting from sand clocks to speed of light ..
Time was the first observation of human after watching sun rise and set . appearing and disappearing of the moon , movement of planets and moving of the stars even.
The book has five chapters describing main elements of time , the metaphysical journey of the sun "amduat" , the year, the months , the days , and eventually the nights.

Pros & Cones: Articles & Short Stories

Pros for four articles; squeezing mind thoughts .
Cones for four pine cones;fantasy love stories.

1736: Part I

Metaphysical Poems , were set as songs lyrics .

6261 Part Ii: Metaphysical Poems

Daily experiences written as song lyrics . all questions that run in mind , emotions in the heart. Struggle of self and conscience and victory in it. In addition There are also some romantic songs.

1735 Part Ii

daily experiences set on papers.. songs .. poetry ... philosophy ..